Fruit Infused Water:

Revitalizing Vitamin Water Recipes - Lose Weight, Detox, And Improve Your Health

© **Copyright 2016 - All rights reserved.**

In no way is it legal to reproduce, duplicate, or transmit any part of this document in either electronic means or in printed format. Recording of this publication is strictly prohibited and any storage of this document is not allowed unless with written permission from the publisher. All rights reserved.

The information provided herein is stated to be truthful and consistent, in that any liability, in terms of inattention or otherwise, by any usage or abuse of any policies, processes, or directions contained within is the solitary and utter responsibility of the recipient reader. Under no circumstances will any legal responsibility or blame be held against the publisher for any reparation, damages, or monetary loss due to the information herein, either directly or indirectly.

Respective authors own all copyrights not held by the publisher.

Legal Notice:

This book is copyright protected. This is only for personal use. You cannot amend, distribute, sell, use, quote or paraphrase any part or the content within this book without the consent of the author or copyright owner. Legal action will be pursued if this is breached.

Disclaimer Notice:

Please note the information contained within this document is for educational and entertainment purposes only. Every attempt has been made to provide accurate, up to date and reliable complete information. No warranties of any kind are expressed or implied. Readers acknowledge that the author is not engaging in the rendering of legal, financial, medical or professional advice.

By reading this document, the reader agrees that under no circumstances are we responsible for any losses, direct or indirect, which are incurred as a result of the use of information contained within this document, including, but not limited to, —errors, omissions, or inaccuracies.

Table of Contents

Introduction 1

Chapter 1: Why Do People Drink Fruit Infused Water? 3

    What is fruit infused water? 3

    Why is fruit infused water the best drink? 4

    How would you start with this? 5

    Benefits of Fruit Infused water 7

        You start consuming more nutrients 7

        You can boost your immunity 7

        You will be able to slow the aging process 7

        You can boost your metabolism 8

        You will be able to rid the excess body weight 8

        You will have more energy than ever before! 8

        A new addition to your diet 8

        Any other health benefits 9

Chapter 2: Benefits of Water and Fruit 10

    Benefits of water 10

    Benefits of Fruit 12

Chapter 3: The Dos and Don'ts! 15

    How do you make fruit infused water? 16

Chapter 4: Recipes for Fruit Infused Water 19

    Apple infused Water recipes 19

        Apple, Cucumber and Ginger Fusion Fruit Infusion water 19

        Apple and Raspberry Fruit Infused Water 20

        Apple and Cinnamon Spa Water Fruit infused Water 21

Apple and Cucumber Fruit Infused Water 22
Blackberry Fruit Infused Water Recipes 23
Blackberry and pear fruit infused water 23
Blueberry Infused Water Recipes 23
Blueberries and Orange Fruit water 23
Creepy fruit infused water 24
Rhubarb Infused Water recipes 25
Cinnamon Rhubarb Explosion 25
Strawberry Infused Water Recipes 26
Strawberries & Mint 26
Strawberry, Kiwi and Parsley Water 27
Cucumber Infused Water Recipes 28
Cucumber & Lemon Medley 28
Citrus Cucumber Water 29
Other Blends 30
Cherry Limeade 30
Pineapple & Mint Medley 30
Zesty Lime and Grapefruit Water 31
Melon, Grape, and Honey Infusion 32
Tropical Coconut and Pineapple Water 33
Raspberry and Thyme Fusion 34
Cranberry and Beet Water 35
Blueberry Chia Water 36
Apricot and Purple Basil Water 37
Black Forrest Cake Water 38
Plum and Persimmon Delight 39
Passion Fruit Fresca 40
Bloody Mary Infusion 41
Blueberry, Cucumber, and Cilantro Water 42
Berry and Sage Water 43
Peach Cobbler Water 44
Lemon Poppy Seed Infusion 45

Dragon Fruit and Grape Water 46

Chapter 5: Healthy Fruit Infused Water Concoction 48

Citrus & Cucumber Water 48

Watermelon and coconut cooler 49

Peach Plum and Pear Infusion 50

Lemon Ginger detox water 51

Blackberry and Orange drink 52

Blueberry and lavender drink 53

Belly slimmer Strawberry and Basil drink 54

Lemon and Berry detox water 55

Watermelon Rosemary Water 57

Strawberry, Apple and Cinnamon drink for beautiful skin 58

Anxiety reliever Pineapple Strawberry drink 59

Blackberry and Sage water 60

Kiwi lemonade 61

Peach and Ginger infused cooler 62

Peach and Ginger Water 63

Cucumber and Lavender Water 64

Grapefruit, Mint & Ginger concoction 65

Papaya and lime concoction 67

Mango and Mint cooler 68

Orange vanilla infused water 69

Cucumber and Jalapeno drink 70

Pineapple and Thyme water 71
Cranberry and Rosemary drink 72
Cranberry, Orange & Bay leaf Cooler 73
Apple and Ginger concoction 74
Cherry and Mint infused Water 75
Mango & lemon grass infused Water 77
Blackberry and Lemon grass infused water 78
Raspberry Peach and Kiwi water 79
Lime and Tarragon detox water 80
Banana Honey and Basil infused water 81
Banana Pineapple and Mint infused water 83
Banana Strawberry & Cardamom infused water 84
Guava and Mango infused water 85
Passion fruit Sage and honey infused water 86
Passion fruit Rosemary and Chia Water 87
Passion fruit and Kiwi infused water 89
Passion fruit, Tender Coconut and Vanilla water 90
Passion fruit, Papaya and Mint infused water 91
Passion fruit Blueberry and cinnamon water 92
Lychee and pineapple infused water 94
Lychee Orange and chia seeds water 95
Lychee and ginger infused water 96
Dragon Fruit coconut water and basil concoction 97
Dragon fruit lemonade 98
Dragon Rosemary and Watermelon drink 100

    Pomegranate and Cucumber drink 101

    Pomegranate Ginger and Limewater 102

Conclusion **104**

Introduction

In this fast paced world, people do not have the time to stop and take a deep breath. They barely have the time to look at how their lives had turned out. But, take a minute and think to yourself whether or not you have achieved all you wanted to in this life. If you tell yourself that you have then you are the luckiest person on this planet! But, the truth is that there are times when you find yourself wanting to get out of the monotony of life and to get rid of all the pent up stress and emotion within you. To be very honest, you will barely find the time to do this, is it not? This is where you have to tell yourself that you are not taking care of yourself! Only when you do this will you be able to live life the way you want to!

When you take a glance around you, you will find that there are people all around you who are on the verge of being obese. This is because of the fact that people do not have the time to take care of themselves due to their respective schedules. But, the one thing they have forgotten is that obesity id the root cause to various health issues which can prove dangerous to you! The lovely fact is that you can get rid of all this by making the tiniest changes to your lifestyle and diet. The concern now is how you will be able to manage this when you have such a tight schedule! Well, this book leaves you with the best thing ever – Fruit Infused Water! The name says everything you need to know about this – you have fruit and you have water too, what more do you need? These two are extremely important in a diet!

You may have been told to drink a lot of water and would have decided that it is the most boring thing to do since it has no flavor to offer! But, when you drink water with the lovely taste of the fruits, you would begin to enjoy consuming a lot of water! This is better than choosing to drink a can of soda, which would never help you reduce weight. This is a great alternative for you when compared to the soda and the other energy drinks that you consume. You will be able to get that surge of energy that you desperately need through a soda or an energy drink, but is that surge enough? You would need more of that surge every hour! You could instead choose an option like fruit infused water, which would leave you healthy!

This book explains to you about fruit infused water and also leaves you with the benefits in order to push you towards that direction. You will see that this water helps you reduce your weight and also helps you detox your body relieving your body off any harmful antibodies! You will find that there are numerous companies that have begun to produce fruit infused water, but why would you want to spend your money on something you can make at home? This book leaves you with numerous recipes that have been explained in detail.

Thank you for purchasing the book. I truly hope you enjoy it.

Chapter 1:
Why Do People Drink Fruit Infused Water?

Before I answer this question, I am going to tell you what fruit infused water is.

What is fruit infused water?

When you had entered a spa for the very first time, were you presented with a tiny glass of water, which when sipped tasted like fruit? That is the fruit infused water that this book will tell you all about! At the end of the book, you will accept that this fruit infused water is a tall glass that helps in refreshing and nourishing you. The best part about drinking fruit infused water is that you can make it at home!

When you have come back from a tough day at work or have finished your chores for the day, you are craving for something to soothe your thirst. You will reach out to a glass of water, but skip it at times since it does not offer any taste. This is when you can use fruit infused water since you will be able to revitalize your body. You know that there is no drink on the face of the planet that can replace water. Mix that up with the vitamins and minerals that the fruits provide you when consumed, and you have the best combination ever – fruit infused water! This water is a lovely blend that has all the elements that you would need. The best part about fruit infused water is that you can add any herbs to give you that burst of flavor! This is healthy and is the most inexpensive drink you could ever come across. You will learn the different benefits that you will obtain through consuming fruit infused water. Let us now understand why it is best that you drink fruit infused water.

Why is fruit infused water the best drink?

The reason we must drink water is to stay hydrates. Another advantage of drinking water is that we can avoid eating excess food. However, many a time people find that water is bland to taste and they might get bored of it. Sometimes people just do not enjoy drinking plain water because of the taste. Hence, people resort to caffeinated drinks or aerated drinks that have adverse effects on a person. However, we can quench our thirst without resorting to either these drinks or water. The healthiest and one of the tastiest solutions to this problem is fruit infused or herb infused water. They are simple to prepare and are also quite healthy. It is not always sweet but is extremely refreshing. These drinks are flavorful and are effective in quenching thirst.

In essence, the process of infusing water is just crushing herbs or fruits and mixing them with water to fuse the flavors. It is definitely a healthier substitute to water than aerated drinks that have high amounts of sugar. Another advantage is that you can pick the flavor that you would like and infuse the water accordingly.

Many people believe that drinking 8 glasses of water a day helps with weight loss. However, it is not easy to have 8 glasses a day. So, you can drink infused water instead. It has the same effect with weight loss. Also, because you will probably infuse the water with flavors you are fond of, drinking 8 glasses of it will not be that difficult.

How would you start with this?

The method of infusing water is quite simple. In theory, it is possible to infuse any flavor into the water. There are many recipes that you could follow. These recipes will involve equipment like infusion bottles and pitchers, blenders. They include a wide array of ingredients as well. Most people prefer to keep the procedure as simple as possible. Since it is literally a substitute for water, it is advisable to keep the preparation procedure simple. Think about any common fruit or vegetable that you like and infuse it. You can also add herbs and spices to the water. You can literally think of any combination and infuse water.

The simplest of recipes to infuse water involve very few ingredients and take about a minute or two. You will have to pick an infusion jar or pitcher, which is basically the container in which you will make your infused water.

The more modern infuser bottles have been designed to make the process of infusion easy. However, they might prove to be slightly on the expensive side. Only purchase them if you wish to consume infused water on a daily basis. Otherwise, a normal container, which you will find at home, will work just fine. The only issue is that the process might get a little dirty and you will have to clean up after. You can use a variety of equipment to mash the herbs, fruits and vegetables. A mortar and pestle or a muddler will do the trick.

The ingredients generally include water; fruits, vegetables, herbs and very rarely they even include spices. The choice of the fruit, vegetable, herb and spice is entirely up to you. You can choose them according to your preferences. However, it is not advisable to use bananas because their texture is rather firm and it may be hard to crush them. The process becomes extremely messy. You must make sure that the fruits are soft and ripe. This will ensure that the flavor of the infused water will be good. The most common fruits used for infusion are citrus fruits and berries because they are quite refreshing. Many people also use pineapples and watermelons because of their sweetness. When it comes to vegetables cucumber is most commonly used. Add ice to your recipe as well. Also include an herb or spice to liven things up.

Once you have decided on your ingredients, you can finally move on to making the infused water. The process more or less stays the same. In case you are making a large amount of infused water, use a jug or pitcher. You can use an infuser bottle for smaller amounts. Fill it up with water. Add the chopped fruits, vegetables, herbs and spices that you have picked. Make sure that they are chopped into small pieces for easier infusion. Another method that you could follow is to puree your ingredients. Pass this puree through a sieve to acquire only the liquid part. Dilute this with water to obtain your infused water.

You will need a lot of patience for this process. You will have to let the mixture to sit for around 8 or 9 hours so that the flavors can get infused properly. The longer you let it sit, the more flavorful the final product will be. Some ingredients infuse quicker when compared to others. Citrus fruits are believed to infuse the fastest. Herbs, on the other hand, can take quite a few hours. Berries also take a long time but they also release pigments that color the water.

Place the infused water in the fridge. When you are serving it, add some ice to enhance its refreshing effect.

Benefits of Fruit Infused water

Have you ever tasted fruit infused water before? This beverage is not only tasty and refreshing but it also has a number of health benefits. Squeeze the fruit a bit before adding it to the infuser pitcher for steeping. This will enhance its nutritional value. There are tons of different recipes and each one has its own benefits.

Given below are a few of the health benefits of fruit infused water:

You start consuming more nutrients

When you infuse water with fruits and other substances, all the nutrients from them get infused as well. Hence, infused water not only tastes better but is also loaded with vitamins, nutrients, minerals and antioxidants. It is clearly a much healthier alternative to energy drinks, aerated drinks and caffeinated drinks.

You can boost your immunity

As you already know, different fruits help in fighting different types of diseases. Therefore, depending on the ingredients that you use, infused water can help in fighting various diseases ranging from cardiovascular diseases to neural illnesses. The components of fruits help in regulating the pH level of the body and this in turn reduces the risks of cancer.

You will be able to slow the aging process

As mentioned earlier, fruit infused water contains antioxidants. They help in slowing down the aging process. Another advantage is that the antioxidants increase the production of collagen that improves skin quality and makes it smooth and silky. It helps you feel younger.

You can boost your metabolism

Fruits have certain compounds in them that help in speeding up metabolism, which in turn causes you to burn more calories. One of the best fruit infused drinks for this purpose is lemon infused water. It promotes the loss of weight.

You will be able to rid the excess body weight

When compared to normal water, fruit infused water is said to be more filling and nutritious. It has lesser calories and sugar than soft drinks and caffeinated drinks. Some fruits also have the effect of reducing your appetite and hence you do not overeat. Hence, by drinking fruit infused water you can have greater control on your weight and you will also stop snacking in between meals.

You will have more energy than ever before!

Since fruit infused drinks are so nutritious, they provide us with large amounts of energy. Hence, it is very effective for athletes, sportspersons and people who go to the gym regularly. In fact, people believe that these drinks can replace sports drinks entirely. In addition to being a healthier alternative, these drinks taste way better than sports drinks.

A new addition to your diet

Fruit infused drinks add variety to your diet. You can come up with any combination of fruits, vegetables, herbs and spices. Since you can always experiment with the taste, it never gets boring and livens up your daily diet.

Any other health benefits

Infused water helps the body with digestion and also helps with other issues in the stomach. As mentioned earlier, these drinks can also help with weight loss. They energize you and leave you feeling refreshed. They also help in cleansing the various systems of the body and have a cooling effect on your stomach.

By now you are aware of the various health benefits of fruit infused drinks. In addition to the health benefits, they are delicious. When you start drinking these drinks you will need to use the basic recipes. Later on, when you are familiar with the process, you can employ more complex recipes for better taste.

Chapter 2:
Benefits of Water and Fruit

In the last chapter, you had gathered the information that you needed about fruit infused water. You were also told about the different benefits that you would obtain on consuming the water. But, why is it that you are asked only to mix fruits in water?

Benefits of water

Water is the best part of every person's diet since it has numerous benefits, which help you, clean your system up! This section covers the benefits of water that will help in reinforcing your belief.

- Water is the best way to flush out any toxins that you may have in your body. It is because of this that you are asked to drink a lot of water so that you will be able to get rid of toxins that are soluble in water. You will be able to remove any minerals or nutrients that may have accumulated in the wrong areas of your body.

- You may have noticed that your body has started to heat up and your cheeks are warm after you have exercised. It is the same when it comes to the changes in weather. This is when water works wonders. It helps in regulating the temperature of your body. You will also be able to replenish all the water you lost through sweat.

- It is good for you to drink water when you are looking at obtaining healthy skin. You will find that it works better than any other cosmetic that claims to clean your face off the acne or the spots and scars. You will find that your skin has achieved a glow that it never had before when you consume a lot of water.

- Water works well in lubricating your muscles and joints and also reduces the friction between the joints. When you consume little or no water, you will find that you have unbearable cramps.

- You will find yourself highly energetic since water helps in creating a balance in the fluids that are found in your body. You will find yourself agile and alert when you are hydrated well.

- Water works wonders when it comes to increasing your metabolic rates. It helps in the quick digestion of food, which would ensure that you never suffer from constipation.

- You will find that you rarely get migraines and headaches that may have been caused by dehydration.

- Water is an essential component that is important for you when you are looking at losing weight. When you are dehydrated, your body has a lower rate of synthesis of proteins that make your body store a lot more calories that leads to a gain in your weight. This is often confused with hunger which makes you eat more when in reality all your body needs is water.

- When you have diarrhea or dysentery, you will lose a lot of fluid that needs to be replenished. If you do not replenish the water, you will be leading yourself towards graver consequences.

It is because of this that it is good for men to drink close to 6 to 8 glasses of water every day while women have to drink a minimum of 5 to 6 glasses every day. You do not have to stick to this measurement and can drink as much water as possible. The following are a few tips that you could use as goals!

- Make sure that you drink a glass of water before every meal. This will ensure that you do not over eat since you will be full. You will also be able to ensure that you stay hydrated.

- Make sure that you carry a bottle of water with you wherever it is that you are going.

- If you find yourself feeling hungry, you can drink water to quench that hunger. You will also be able to avoid the additional calories that you may gain.

- Make sure that you have a jug that is filled with the fruit infused water in the fridge to make sure that you drink this whenever you find it difficult to make one glass of the fruit infused water if you are in a hurry.

Benefits of Fruit

Fruits are an important component of a diet and are very important since they nourish your body and also provide it with nutrients that are vital for your health and in the maintenance of your body.

- Certain fruits – bananas, peaches and prunes – help in the maintenance of the blood pressure since they are rich in potassium.

- It is important that you consume fruits that are rich in fiber since they help in reducing any cholesterol in your blood and also reduce the risk of procuring heart diseases. These fruits help in improving the function of your bowels and also leave you with a feeling of fullness that results in the fact that you do not feel hungry that often.

- The calories in fruits are very less in number and even if they are present, they are healthy and needed by your body.

- Folic acid in fruits helps in improving the formation of the blood cells in your body. It is important that pregnant women consume these fruits. This also helps in reducing the possibility of ailments like the defects of neural tubes.

- It is important that you consume fruits with vitamin C in them since they help in the growth of the tissues in your body thereby healing any wounds.

- When you have a lot of fruits in your diet, you will find that you have a reduced risk of procuring diabetes and cardiovascular diseases.

- Fruits help in keeping your eyes healthy and they also help in preventing any eye diseases that may be related to your age.

It is for these very reasons that it is important that you consume a diet that is rich in fruits. There are a few tips you could use when it comes to eating more fruits as a part of your diet.

1. You will need to ensure that you purchase a good amount of fruits when you go to the supermarket. You can always choose to purchase frozen or canned fruits.

2. Make sure that you have a bowl of fruit placed on your coffee and dining tables to ensure that you are motivated to eat one of these fruits.

3. Make sure that you cut up some fruit and leave it in the refrigerator in order to consume it later.

4. Make sure that you add a few fruits to your meals. You could add fruits to your cereal or have a fruit right before you begin eating a meal. You could also have a fruit salad.

5. If you are hungry, you can eat fruit instead of consuming any junk food.

6. Make sure that you eat dry fruits if you cannot have fresh fruits. But, you have to ensure that you consume much lesser of the dry fruits when compared to the fresh fruit.

Chapter 3:
The Dos and Don'ts!

When you are back from work on a day when it is hot, you may choose to consume a can of soda or carbonated drinks. It is true that these drinks do nothing but cause harm to your body. The sodas that have claimed to be diet sodas are worse than the regular sodas and have to be avoided like the plague. These sodas contain a lot of artificial sweeteners that cause numerous diseases.

When you consume a diet soda, you will find that you have not lost weight but have gained weight instead. You may have been under the impression that you will obtain a surge of energy, which is true, but it is also true that you will be giving your body a dose of sugar that leads to diabetes and heart diseases. It has been shown that your teeth also tend to deteriorate when you consume too much of the soda. The soda causes the teeth to lose their calcium content leaving them soft.

When you continue to drink the sodas, you will find that your body has begun to crave more for the sodas leaving you in a cycle that is harmful to you! When you purchase any flavored water at the supermarket, you will find that there are a lot of additives that have large amounts of sugar, which lead to diabetes. Flavored water is better than the sodas but they do not do much help either. You can therefore choose to be fresh and hydrated by consuming fruit infused water that you have made at home! You will be very glad to know that this water has no additives since you will be making it yourself! You will be able to detox your body as well and will be able to rid your body of any toxins!

You may choose to consume coffee every morning to wake yourself up to gear yourself up for the day. You will not be hurt too much by the coffee but there is the drug, caffeine, which is harmful for you. Your body will be harmed too much by the drug. If you consume too much coffee you will find yourself nauseous and will also have heart palpitations. You will need to therefore, consider every sip of coffee you take. It is best to choose fruit infused water since you will be able to keep yourself fresh and happy.

How do you make fruit infused water?

You may have been experimenting with numerous techniques to lose weight and to also stay healthy. But, this method is the simplest way to lose weight too! You can follow the steps given below when you are looking at making your very own fruit infused water.

Step 1

You will need to decide what kind of fruit infused water you want and why you are choosing that particular type. Now, gather the fruits and place the fruits in a jug full of water and ice. Store it in the refrigerator. You will need to follow the certain rules when it comes to the same:

- Use fruits that are ripe and fresh in order to obtain the best flavor of the fruit.

- Make sure that you have certain herbs which will ensure that you can make the water much better.

- Make sure that you use jars when you are making the fruit infused water. Make sure that you have mason jars which have been decorated well when it comes to serving guests the water.

- You could also choose to purchase certain fruit infusion bottles since that will help you carry the water all around with you.

- You could use a wooden spoon in order to mix the ingredients well together and to extract the juice from the fruit.

Step 2

You will need to add cold water to the pitcher and ensure that the water that you have in the pitcher is the same amount that you want.

Step 3

You can add how many ever ice cubes you would want to.

Step 4

You have to slice the fruits up into the size that you have chosen in order to add only the required amount of fruit to the water. You do not want to make a pulpy drink and will need to ensure that you have the right quantity of fruit.

Step 5

You will need to bruise the fruits a little in order to ensure that the fruit has infused into the water.

Step 6

You will need to shake the pitcher in order to give the water a taste. If you find that the flavor is the right amount you will have to cut up more fruit in order to ensure that the flavor is according to your taste. If you find that you need to add a little sugar, avoid that since it is best to add natural syrups like maple syrup or honey. You will then have to leave it in the refrigerator for a few hours.

Step 7

You will need to pour the water into glasses and serve it with a little garnish with a few herbs. Now drink it up! You have your very own fruit infused water! You can do this with any fruit you would want since you will be able to obtain different benefits. There are some that may boost your energy while there are others that work towards boosting your metabolism or your immunity by flushing out the toxins.

Chapter 4: Recipes for Fruit Infused Water

Apple infused Water recipes

Apple, Cucumber and Ginger Fusion Fruit Infusion water

This infused water infused with apple, cucumber and ginger is extremely effective in increasing your metabolism and it is hence advisable to consume it when you have overeaten. It will also keep you hydrated and increases your stamina. It can also help with weight loss.

Apples are quite filling and so this drink will make sure you do not keep snacking on junk food and this helps in controlling your weight. The cucumbers help in flushing out the toxins in your body and keep you hydrated. The ginger helps in enhancing your metabolism and also increases your energy levels (stamina).

Ingredients

- 2 – 3 slices of apple
- 2 slices of cucumber
- Piece of chopped ginger

Instructions

- Place the ingredients in a bowl and mix them.
- Now place this mixture into an Aqua blend basket.

- Add water into the basket.
- Leave this mixture in the fridge for some time to get maximum refreshment.

Apple and Raspberry Fruit Infused Water

To have good health, good digestion is an absolute must. However, fighting digestive troubles is not simple. Apple and raspberry infused water is a drink that can help fight these issues though. The raspberries have more fiber than most fruits and have low sugar content. They also have very few calories. Hence, they are good for people with diabetes and also for those who are looking to lose weight. The apples on the other hand have pectin, which helps in detoxifying the body and also aids in digestion.

Ingredients

- 3 slightly squeezed raspberries
- 3 thin slices of apple

Instructions

- Take an Aqua blend basket. Place the apples and raspberries in it.
- Fill it up with water and mix it a little bit.
- Let the mixture stand for at least an hour for infusion to take place.
- If you infuse it overnight, it will enhance the taste of the drink.

- Once all the drink has been consumed, you can eat the fruit that has been left behind.

Apple and Cinnamon Spa Water Fruit infused Water

This drink helps in increasing the energy levels of a person. It also helps in increasing stamina. This drink is extremely tasty and regulates the blood sugar level as well. Here is the recipe to make apple and cinnamon spa water infused water. This drink is the best since the apple used contains numerous antioxidants like Vitamin C and cinnamon contains the property where it can regulate the blood sugar levels thereby preventing diabetes. You will also be able to reduce the pain that is caused due to arthritis. When you work, you will find yourself much more efficient and focused.

Ingredients

- 4 thinly sliced Apple (halved)
- ½ Cinnamon stick

Instructions

- Take a container and mix the ingredients together.
- Now take this mixture and place it in an Acquablend bottle.
- Fill the entire bottle with water.
- Let it rest in the fridge for around 2 hours so that the flavors and nutrients get infused.

Apple and Cucumber Fruit Infused Water

One major advantage of apple and cucumber infused water is weight loss. Apples have various health benefits and improve your overall health. Cucumbers have a large fiber content which helps in digestion. It can also help with other stomach-related issues.

Ingredients

- 3 slices apple, halved
- 3 slices cucumber, halved

Instructions

- Mix the apple halves and cucumber halves in a container.
- Place them into an Acquablend basket making sure that they are in equal amounts.
- Make sure that you do not fill more than 2/3 of the basket with fruit
- Now fill it up with water until the brim.
- Leave this mixture in the fridge for at least an hour or two to allow for the process of infusion to take place.
- You can choose to let it stay in the refrigerator through the night for greater flavor.

Blackberry Fruit Infused Water Recipes

Blackberry and pear fruit infused water

There are many berries and fruits that are specific to the autumn season. You can enjoy all these fruits with this drink. It mainly includes blackberries and pears. Blackberries have low amounts of fat and calories. According to recent studies, they also help in improving cognitive skills. Pears also have their own benefits. They aid in managing your weight.

Ingredients

- 4 Blackberries
- 2 pear slices, quartered

Instructions

- Take an Acquablend basket and place the berries and pear slices in it.
- Now fill it up with water.
- Let it rest in the fridge for a few hours for infusion. Leave it in the fridge overnight for stronger flavors.

Blueberry Infused Water Recipes

Blueberries and Orange Fruit water

This drink has a ton of health advantages. It is known to boost a person's immune system. Blueberries are also believed to have certain healing properties that are very effective. This drink also improves skin condition and memory power.

Oranges have a large amount of phytonutrients and vitamin C. They also contain decent amounts of various other vitamins. They are rich in minerals such as copper and calcium.

Ingredients

- 5 blueberries

- 2 slices of orange, halved

Instructions

- Take a container and mix the blueberries and orange slices in it.

- Transfer this mixture to an Acquablend bottle.

- Fill the Acquablend bottle with water.

- Let it rest in the fridge for a few hours for infusion. Leave it in the fridge overnight for stronger flavors.

Creepy fruit infused water

This name might seem extremely absurd at first glance. It is a drink that is specially made for Halloween. It is a fun looking drink and is perfect for a Halloween party. In addition to being a party drink, it tastes delicious and is extremely nutritious and comes with a number of health benefits. It consists mainly of lychees and blueberries.

The 2 main components of lychees and blueberries are very rich in vitamin C, which happens to be a natural antioxidant. They also contain fiber and other vitamins that help with digestion and also enhance metabolism of proteins, carbs and fats.

Ingredients

- 2-3 Lychee (peeled and pitted if fresh – or drained from tin)
- 2-3 large blueberries

Instructions

- Remove the seeds from the lychees. Now carefully insert the blueberries into these cavities in order to make something that looks like "eyeballs".
- Put these "eyeballs" into an Acquablend bottle.
- Fill the bottle with water.
- Let it rest in the fridge for a few hours for infusion. Leave it in the fridge overnight for stronger flavors.

Rhubarb Infused Water recipes

Cinnamon Rhubarb Explosion

Rhubarb is highly nutritious. It contains loads of vitamins, minerals, organic compounds and other substances that help keep our body healthy. It also provides us with fiber. It aids us in weight loss and helps prevent cardiovascular illnesses. It increases bone strength and also improves the circulation of blood. Cinnamon also helps by regulating the sugar levels in blood.

Ingredients

- 1 stalk of rhubarb
- 1 small apple
- A stick of cinnamon
- Water

Instructions

- Cut the stalk of rhubarb into big pieces.
- Take the apple and wash it thoroughly. Cut it into thin slices.
- Mix these two ingredients in a container and then transfer them into an infuser bottle. Fill the bottle up with cold water.
- Now leave the mixture in the fridge for a few hours and let infusion take place. It is advisable to leave it overnight. Serve chilled.

Strawberry Infused Water Recipes

Strawberries & Mint

The strawberry in the water will work wonders since it has properties of being an antioxidant and an anti – inflammatory! It works towards preventing your skin from sagging as well!

Ingredients

- 8 Strawberries (medium sized) sliced thin
- 4 sprigs of mint
- ½ quart of water and ice

Instructions

Take an Acquablend bottle and place all the ingredients inside. Add water to it. Let the mixture stand for around an hour for infusion to take place effectively. Serve with ice.

Strawberry, Kiwi and Parsley Water

The ingredients of this drink are extremely tasty. Most people love the taste of kiwis and strawberries. This drink is very refreshing. Kiwis are very rich in vitamins C and E that help in battling cancer, ageing and also boost the immune system. They also contain serotonin that has digestive and cardiovascular functions. Serotonin also helps in regulating our sleep cycles. Kiwis also contain a chemical called lutein. This is a vitamin that combats eye defects that are age related. Strawberries contain anthocyanins that help in reducing unwanted fat. They also promote bone strength and prevent esophageal cancer.

Ingredients

- 1 kiwi
- A cup of strawberries
- A few sprigs of parsley

- Half a lemon

- Water

Instructions

- Wash the kiwi and the lemon thoroughly. Cut them into very thin slices.

- Halve all the strawberries. Place them in a container along with lemon and kiwi. Mix them well.

- Transfer the contents into an infuser bottle. Add the sprigs of parsley. Fill the bottle up with cold water.

- You need not place this in the fridge for infusion, as it tastes good even when at normal temperature. However, it is better to serve the drink with ice.

Cucumber Infused Water Recipes

Cucumber & Lemon Medley

The cucumber in this water works as an anti – inflammatory and also helps in controlling the retention of water! Lemon helps in digestion and also keeps you away from the common cold!

Ingredients

- 3 cups chilled still spring or mineral water

- 6 thin slices of cucumber

- 2 thin slices of lemon

Instructions

Take a container and mix the cucumber and lemon slices in it. Now add the water. Mix it properly. Place in the fridge for at least 2 hours for infusion to take place. Leave overnight for a richer flavor. Serve with ice cubes.

Citrus Cucumber Water

The cucumber in this water works as an anti – inflammatory and also helps in controlling the retention of water! Lemon helps in digestion and also keeps you away from the common cold! The oranges and the limes contain Vitamin C that helps in cleaning your system from the toxins that may have accumulated.

Ingredients

- 2 large lemons, sliced
- 2 large limes, sliced
- 2 large oranges, sliced
- 2 large cucumbers, sliced
- 1 gallon of water

Instructions

Take an infuser bottle and add the lemons, limes, cucumbers and oranges. Fill it up with water. Infuse overnight in the fridge. Add the juice of one orange while serving for richer flavor.

Other Blends

Cherry Limeade

The cherries in the blend and the lime have a high quantity of Vitamin C that acts as a perfect detoxing agent for the body. You will be able to clear your system of any germs or antibodies.

Ingredients

- ½ Key lime, sliced thinly
- 3-pitted cherries cut in half
- ½ sprig of mint

Instructions

Take a container and mix the lime and cherries in it. Fill it up with water. Now add the mint. Place in the fridge over night for the flavors and nutrients to get infused. Serve chilled.

Pineapple & Mint Medley

Pineapple and mint are great ingredients, which need to be consumed more often since you will be able to clear your body of toxins. You will also be able to boost your metabolism and your digestion.

Ingredients

- 2 pineapple slices
- 1 sprig of mint

- ½ quart of water and ice

Instructions

Mix the ingredients in an infusion bottle and fill with water. You need not place this in the fridge for infusion, as it tastes good even when at normal temperature. Serve with ice.

Zesty Lime and Grapefruit Water

This recipe for infused water is extremely refreshing and is perfect for summers. The citrus fruits present in it will provide you with vitamin C and the drink itself will keep you hydrated. You can experiment with a variety of combinations of the citrus fruits and pick them according to your preferences.

Ingredients

- 2 limes
- 1 red grapefruit
- 1 orange
- 1 lemon
- Water

Instructions

- Firstly, you will have to halve the limes, lemon, orange and grapefruit. Now cut these halves into thin slices.
- Now take an infuser bottle or beaker and place all the ingredients in it. Fill it up with water until the brim.

- Now leave the mixture in the fridge and let infusion take place. It is advisable to leave it overnight. Serve chilled.

Melon, Grape, and Honey Infusion

This is another drink that is extremely refreshing and is perfect for a hot day. The honeydew melons are sweet and are rich in B complex vitamins. Green grapes contain large amounts of vitamins and minerals and also have cancer-fighting properties. The honey and mint are not just for adding to the flavor. They have anti-microbial and anti-fungal properties. In addition to these health benefits, the drink tastes absolutely amazing.

Ingredients

- 2 honeydew melon wedges
- 1 cup of green grapes
- Around 15 mint leaves
- Water

Instructions

- Take the honeydew melon wedges and remove the middle part or core. Now cut them up into small pieces.
- Cut the green grapes in half. Place them and the honeydew melon into an infuser bottle.
- Now add the mint leaves as well. Add a small amount of honey for taste. Fill up with water.

- Let the mixture stand for around an hour or two for infusion to take place effectively. Serve with ice.

Tropical Coconut and Pineapple Water

Have you ever tasted a Pina Colada? This drink tastes about the same so it is absolutely delicious. It also has quite a few health benefits. Coconuts are known for their electrolyte content and make this drink extremely refreshing. The pineapple has large amounts of magnesium and ascorbic acid. The drink keeps you hydrated.

Ingredients

- 1 small pineapple
- 1 young coconut
- Half a vanilla bean pod for flavor
- Water

Instructions

- Take the pineapple and cut it down the middle. Remove the core. Now chop up the pineapple into bite-size pieces.
- Now take the coconut. Cut off the top part. Make a hole along the cut portion and pour out the coconut water into a glass (this can be used as a drink by itself). Remove the flesh of the coconut.
- Place all the ingredients in an infuser bottle and mix them a little bit. Now fill it up with water.

- You need not place this in the fridge for infusion, as it tastes good even when at normal temperature. However, it is better to serve the drink with ice.

Raspberry and Thyme Fusion

The components of this drink are extremely rich in vitamins. Raspberries are especially packed with loads of vitamin B7, also known as biotin. Biotin has a number of beauty benefits. It prevents aging, promotes smoother and softer skin, improves strength of hair and also helps in eliminating scars of pimples or acne. The thyme adds a very characteristic flavor to the drink and it also has high iron content.

Ingredients

- 2 cups of raspberries
- 1 cup of baby spinach
- 1 lime
- A few sprigs of thyme
- Water

Instructions

- Firstly, you will need to wash the lime. Now cut it up into thin slices.

- Take an infuser bottle or basket depending on the quantity required (bottle for smaller quantities and basket for larger). Now add the slices of lime, raspberries, cut spinach and thyme into the bottle. Fill the bottle up with cold water

- Place in the fridge for at least 2 hours for infusion to take place. Leave overnight for a richer flavor. Serve with ice cubes.

Cranberry and Beet Water

The main ingredient of this drink is the beetroot. It has a very mild and pleasing taste and is loaded with vitamins. It is especially rich in vitamins A (retinol), C (ascorbic acid) and D (calciferol). It also has a large content of iron and calcium. The cranberries have a tart taste and mix very well with the taste of the beets. This drink keeps you hydrated and is extremely refreshing.

Ingredients

- 1 small beet
- A small amount of beet greens (a handful will do)
- Half a cup of cranberries
- A teaspoon or two of honey for flavor
- Water

Instructions

- Wash the beetroot. Now chop it up into thin slices.
- Take an infuser bottle. Place all the sliced beets, cranberries and beet greens in it. Fill it up with water. Add a small amount of honey. Do not add more than 2 teaspoons or the taste of the drink will be dominated by the honey.

- Leave this mixture in the fridge for at least an hour or two to allow for the process of infusion to take place. You can choose to let it stay in the refrigerator through the night for greater flavor.

Blueberry Chia Water

Chia seeds are said to be able to absorb up to 10 times their weight in water. They are extremely healthy as they are packed with nutrients. These nutrients can have important effects on your body and brain. The seeds have very low calorific content. The health advantages of blueberries have already been stated before. This drink is extremely refreshing and is ideal during summer.

Ingredients

- Half a cup of blueberries
- Around a tablespoon of chia seeds
- One lemon
- A small amount of honey for flavor
- Water

Instructions

- First, take the lemon and wash it. Cut it up into thin slices.
- Take a container and place the blueberries, chia seeds and slices of lemon into it. Mix them well.

- Take an infuser bottle and add these ingredients along with cold water. Add honey making sure that it does not exceed a teaspoon.

- Now leave the mixture in the fridge for a few hours and let infusion take place. It is advisable to leave it overnight. Serve chilled.

Apricot and Purple Basil Water

The main ingredients for this drink, as the name suggests, are apricots and purple basil. Apricots are loaded with antioxidants that help in preventing or fighting cancer. Purple basil is believed to help with the circulation of blood. It can also combat insomnia.

Ingredients

- 2 large apricots
- ½ a naval orange
- Around 10 or 15 purple basil leaves
- Water

Instructions

- Take the apricots. Wash them properly and cut them in half. Remove the pits.

- Wash the oranges. Now cut them up into thin slices.

- Take a big container and mix the apricots and oranges in it. Transfer the contents to an infuser bottle and fill it up with water.

- Let the mixture stand for around an hour or two for infusion to take place effectively. Serve with ice.

Black Forrest Cake Water

For this infused water drink, we use sour cherries, coconuts and dates as the main ingredients. It is inspired by the classic Black Forrest cake. Coconuts are filled with electrolytes and hence this drink is extremely refreshing. The sour cherries have a very particular taste and also help in improving skin health. The dates are sweet and have a taste very similar to that of chocolate but they are rich in minerals such as potassium and magnesium.

Ingredients

- Half a cup of coconut flesh
- Three to four medium dates
- Around 10 sour cherries
- A few drops of liquid stevia
- Water

Instructions

- Take the dates. Cut them in halve and pit them. Do the same with the berries as well.
- Take a container and mix the dates, coconut flesh and berries. Transfer the contents to an infuser bottle and fill it up with cold water.

- Add a few drops of liquid stevia. Place in the fridge for at least 2 hours for infusion to take place. Leave overnight for a richer flavor. Serve with ice cubes.

Plum and Persimmon Delight

Persimmons are highly nutritious fruits that are rich in vitamins, minerals and essential anti-oxidants. Although these are moderately high in calories, they have low fat content. They are very good sources of fiber. Persimmons are especially rich in vitamin A and vitamin C. Purple plums are rich in various minerals such as magnesium, iron and potassium. Bay leaves (an additional ingredient) have a cooling effect on the stomach and also facilitate digestion.

Ingredients

- 2 small persimmons
- 2 purple plums
- A few sprigs of parsley
- 1 bay leaf
- Water

Instructions

- Take the persimmons. Wash and cut them.
- Take the plums and wash them. Pit and halve them. Now take a container and add these to the container along with the persimmons. Mix the ingredients.

- Transfer the contents to an infuser bottle and fill it up with water. Leave this mixture in the fridge for at least an hour or two to allow for the process of infusion to take place. You can choose to let it stay in the refrigerator through the night for greater flavor.

Passion Fruit Fresca

Passion fruit has a very characteristic taste that stands out. It is both sweet and tart to taste. It has a number of health benefits. Some of these benefits include the prevention of cancerous growth, enhancement of immune function, improvement of eyesight, betterment of skin, regulation of blood pressure, enhancement of blood circulation and improved bone density. It also helps in stimulating digestion. The oranges and honey will add taste to the drink and also add to the vitamin C content. Parsley is used to add freshness.

Ingredients

- 1 passion fruit
- 1 naval orange
- A few sprigs of parsley
- Water
- A teaspoon of honey for flavor

Instructions

- Wash the oranges properly. Cut them up into thin slices.

- Now, take the passion fruit and halve it. Remove the insides and add them to a container. To this container add the orange slices as well and mix.

- Transfer the mixture to an infuser bottle and add the honey and parsley. Fill the bottle up with cold water.

- Now leave the mixture in the fridge for a few hours and let infusion take place. It is advisable to leave it overnight. Serve chilled.

Bloody Mary Infusion

Bloody Mary is originally a cocktail of vodka and tomato juice. This infused water drink is inspired by the cocktail. Needless to say, it has a lot less calories than the actual cocktail and does not include alcohol of any form. Tomatoes are a great source of antioxidants and hence help combat cancer. They have the ability to help regulate blood pressure. Tomatoes also have high fiber content and can help prevent constipation. It tastes great and is extremely refreshing.

Ingredients

- 1 tomato (cherry tomatoes will work as well)
- 1 stalk of celery
- A few drops of hot sauce
- A few sprigs of cilantro
- Water

Instructions

- Wash the tomatoes and celery stalk. Cut them up into really thin slices.

- Place these into a container and mix them. Transfer the contents into an infuser bottle and add the sprigs of cilantro. Add a few drops of hot sauce (depending on how spicy you want the drink to be).

- Add cold water to the mixture.

- Let the mixture stand for around an hour or two for infusion to take place effectively. Serve with ice.

Blueberry, Cucumber, and Cilantro Water

Any berry infused water generally tastes great and is extremely refreshing. This drink can also help you to lose weight. The cucumber and cilantro help in boosting metabolism. Blueberries are rich in nutrients and have low calories. They have a very high content of antioxidants. They also protect the cholesterol in the blood and DNA from getting damaged.

Ingredients

- 1 cup of blueberries

- 1 cucumber (preferably a smaller one)

- 1 lemon

- A few sprigs of cilantro

- Water

Instructions

- Wash the lemon and cucumber. Cut them into thin slices.

- Take a container and add the lemon and cucumber slices to it. Transfer these contents into an infuser bottle. Fill it up with cold water and add the berries and cilantro sprigs as well.

- You need not place this in the fridge for infusion, as it tastes good even when at normal temperature. However, it is better to serve the drink with ice.

Berry and Sage Water

Berries are very good sources of antioxidants and hence help in battling cancer. Also, they are extremely refreshing. Sage is an herb that has a number of health benefits. It is very effective in treating digestive problems such as loss of appetite, diarrhea and heartburn. Sage is also highly rich in copper, iron and vitamin B1.

Ingredients

- 1 cup of blueberries

- 1 cup of raspberries

- 1 cup of blackberries

- Around 10 sage leaves

- Water

Instructions

- Wash all the berries thoroughly. Place them in a container.

- Now, add the sage into this container and slightly muddle it with the berries to intensify the flavor. Transfer this mixture into an infuser bottle.

- Fill up the bottle with cold water. Place in the fridge for at least 2 hours for infusion to take place. Leave overnight for a richer flavor. Serve with ice cubes.

Peach Cobbler Water

This drink is inspired by the classic dessert of Peach Cobbler. It combines peaches and coconuts to give a drink that tastes absolutely delicious. A peach is an excellent source of vitamin C (an antioxidant) and can help fight cancer. It also helps in improving overall skin health by making it smoother, removing wrinkles and scars of acne and pimples. It also helps with improving the health of the heart. Peaches are also rich in magnesium and potassium. As mentioned earlier, coconuts are storehouses of electrolytes and are very refreshing.

Ingredients

- 1 peach (ripe)

- 1 young coconut

- A few drops of vanilla liquid stevia drops

- Water

Instructions

- Wash the peaches. Cut them up into very thin slices.

- Cut off the top of the coconut. Make a hole in the cut surface and pour out the water into a container and store that in the fridge (this can be used as a refreshing drink by itself).

- Remove the flesh from the inside of the coconut. Put this flesh in an infuser bottle.

- Also add the peach slices and a few drops of the vanilla stevia. Fill the bottle up with cold water.

- Leave this mixture in the fridge for at least an hour or two to allow for the process of infusion to take place. You can choose to let it stay in the refrigerator through the night for greater flavor.

Lemon Poppy Seed Infusion

When it comes to the cooking industry, the combination of lemon and poppy seed is very common. Lemons have very few calories. They are also rich in pectin fiber, vitamin C, calcium and potassium. They also have antibacterial properties. Lemons are known to maintain the pH level of the blood and also help with digestion by promoting the production of bile. Poppy seeds are excellent sources of B complex vitamins. Poppy seeds are rich in minerals like iron, copper, calcium, potassium, zinc and magnesium.

Ingredients

- 1 lemon
- A few poppy seeds (around 1 teaspoon)
- 1 or 2 teaspoons of honey
- 4 mint leaves
- Water

Instructions

- Wash the lemons properly. Cut them up into very thin slices.
- Take the slices in a container and add the mint leaves and poppy seeds. Mix them properly. Transfer the contents of the container to an infuser bottle. Now add the honey and fill the bottle up with cold water.
- Let the mixture stand for around an hour or two for infusion to take place effectively. Squeeze the juice of a lemon in while serving to intensify the flavor. Serve with ice.

Dragon Fruit and Grape Water

The dragon fruit is extremely appealing to the eye due to its neon color. In addition to looking really good, the dragon fruit is highly nutritious. For starters, it has low amounts of cholesterol. It has decent amounts of dietary fiber and antioxidants. It also helps in fighting diabetes and ageing of the skin. The fruit also suppresses arthritis. The main health benefit of red grapes is that they clean up any brain damaging plaque. In addition to this, they protect the heart and promote weight loss.

Ingredients

- 1 pink dragon fruit
- A cup of red grapes
- 1 small cucumber
- Around 10 mint leaves
- Water

Instructions

- Wash the red grapes thoroughly. Halve them once they are dry.
- Peel the dragon fruit carefully. Cut the fruit into large chunks.
- Wash the cucumbers as well. Cut them into thin slices. Transfer the slices into a container and add the dragon fruit and grapes. Mix them a bit and transfer these contents into an infuser bottle and add water and mint leaves.
- Place in the fridge for at least 2 hours for infusion to take place. Leave overnight for a richer flavor. Serve with ice cubes.

Chapter 5: Healthy Fruit Infused Water Concoction

Citrus & Cucumber Water

Most of us find it difficult to get through the summer heat without indulging in fizzy drinks. The humidity could get overwhelming especially if you stay in a tropical country. Citrus fruits like oranges and lemon contain a high amount of vitamin C, which could detoxify the liver as well as the digestive tract. The enzymes present in citrus fruits also help in increasing your metabolism, thus breaking down the fat in your body. Cucumber on the other hand acts as an anti-inflammatory agent, thereby keeping your skin hydrated.

Ingredients

- 2 fresh oranges (sliced)
- Approximately 10 cups of regular water
- 1 lemon
- 1 medium cucumber (sliced)
- 4-5 mint leaves

Instructions

- Slice up the lemons
- Put the sliced lemons, oranges and cucumber in a large pitcher along with the mint leaves. Mix them properly.

- Add 10 cups of water to the pitcher and mix well again using a large spoon.

- Place the pitcher in the refrigerator for a minimum of 3 hours for the infusion process to take place. Leaving it in the fridge overnight brings a rich flavor to it. Serve in large glasses with some ice cubes in it.

Watermelon and coconut cooler

Watermelon being naturally refreshing feels extremely soothing amidst the scorching summer heat. High on anti oxidants, watermelon is known to be helpful in avoiding obesity or heart diseases. Besides the health benefits, water melon also keeps your skin hydrated for a long time and also helps in promoting a healthy glow on the face. Also, coconut acts as a cooling agent while being high on fiber and essential minerals. A perfect combination of sweet and refreshing taste, this pink cooler is sure to become a staple in your house.

Ingredients

- 4 cups of de-seeded and cubed watermelon
- 4 cups of coconut water
- 7-8 cups of regular water
- 1 sliced lemon

Instructions

- Place the cubed watermelon into an infuser.

- To it, add the coconut water, regular water and mix well.

- Cut lemon slices and add them to the infuser. Stir well for about a minutes.

- Let the mixture stand for a minimum of two hours for the infusion to take place. For better results leave it overnight in the refrigerator. Serve along with ice cubes.

Peach Plum and Pear Infusion

As titillating as it sounds to your taste buds, this relishing drink is sure to keep you fresh all day. Peaches are a rich source of vitamin A, potassium and iron. On the other hand, plums contain a high amount of fiber and sorbitol. The vitamin A present in peaches and plums are highly useful for human eyesight. Pears are often recommended by dieticians for weight loss or for curing digestive issues. They also aid against risk of developing colon cancer.

Ingredients

- 2 medium sized peaches

- 2 small plums

- 2 pears

- 9-10 cups of water

- 4 leaves of mint

Instructions

- Wash and slice the peaches, plums, and pears and set them aside in a bowl.

- Transfer these slices to a large infuser along with the mint leaves. Mix them well. Add 3 10 cups of water to the infuser and stir well for about a minute.

- Let this mixture stand for about 2 hours before serving. Alternatively, you can store it in the refrigerator for about 24 hours. Serve the drink with ice cubes.

Lemon Ginger detox water

The increasing rate of obesity issues in recent times causes people to go overboard with weight loss diets. While most weight loss products are being sold at outrageous prices in the market, a combination of lemon and ginger is highly effective as well as light on your pockets. Ginger, often used for weight loss is also loaded with gingerols, a cleansing agent that contains anti cancer properties. The zesty lemon helps in flushing out toxins from your body, while adding a refreshingly tangy flavor to your drink. This vibrant drink is also a surefire way to refresh yourself quickly without adding a lot of calories to your diet.

Ingredients

- 7-8 cups of water

- 1 medium sized ginger root (sliced or grated)

- 1 lemon

- 4 mint leaves

- 2 tablespoons of honey

Instructions

- Wash the lemon and cut thin slices

- Add the slices to an infuser along with sliced ginger root and mint leaves. Mix well.

- Add 7-8 cups of water to the infuser honey and stir well for a minute. Let the mixture stand for 2-3 hours before you serve, so it infuses well. Storing this drink in the refrigerator for 24hours gives it a richer flavor. Add ice cubes while serving.

Blackberry and Orange drink

These two super foods, blackberry and orange, make for a wonderful concoction of flavors while being loaded with abundance of healing agents. Packed with a high amount of vitamin C, they are extremely delightful in flavor. Regular intake of oranges and blackberries can keep your immune system strengthened and does wonders to your skin. Oranges are considered to be one of the healthiest fruits that can boost your energy levels quickly. Colorful and rich in flavors, this concoction can also keep ulcers at bay.

Ingredients

- 7-8 cups of regular water
- 2 mandarin oranges
- 1 cup blackberries

Instructions

- Wash the oranges properly and cut them into thin slices.
- Add these slices to an infuser along with blackberries. Mix them well. Add some water to this mixture and stir it well.
- When you let this mixture stand for 2-3 hours, it shall infuse well.
- To extract richness of the fruits, store it in the fridge overnight. Serve the drink along with ice cubes. You can also relish on the fruit slices after you have consumed the drink.

Blueberry and lavender drink

When it comes to fruit infused detox water, we want to make sure to keep it interesting. A daily dose of the same detox drink can get boring and take the fun out of the detox diet. Lavender petals can add a wonderful yet subtle floral aroma to an otherwise boring detox drink. At the same time, it is known to have anti-inflammatory and antiseptic properties. Combine this with the highly hydrating blueberries and you have an amazing concoction that makes your skin radiant while flushing out all the bad toxins from the body.

Ingredients

- 1 cup fresh blueberries
- A handful of edible lavender petals
- About 7-8 cups of water

Instructions

- Wash the blueberries properly.
- Take a large infuser and add the blueberries as well as lavender petals to it. Ensure that the lavender petals are fresh and properly cleaned.
- Mix this drink well by stirring it for about a minute.
- Leave this drink aside for a good 3 hours for the infusion process to take place. A richer aroma can be obtained by leaving this mixture in the refrigerator for a whole day. Always serve it with ice cubes.

Belly slimmer Strawberry and Basil drink

Curbing your appetite can seem like an uphill task, especially when you are on a weight loss diet. The frequent hunger pangs can send you into a frenzy, making it difficult to concentrate on your daily tasks. Regular use of basil in your diet can leave you feeling fuller and energized throughout the day. An upset tummy, frequent hunger pangs, and fluid retention can all be taken care of by using basil in your detox drink. Also, a handful of strawberries could add a nice flavor to the drink while providing a high amount of fiber essential for weight loss.

Ingredients

- 4 basil leaves

- 6-7 freshly picked strawberries (sliced)

- Half a cucumber (sliced)

- 10-12 cups of water

Instructions

- Wash the basil leaves and roughly chop them.

- In an infuser, put the strawberry and cucumber slices along with the basil leaves and mix them well.

- Add some water to this mixture and stir well using a large spoon. It is necessary to let this mixture stand for 3 hours for it to infuse well. Similarly, you can store this mixture in the refrigerator and drink it at least twice a day.

- Serve this drink in a large glass with a few ice cubes.

Lemon and Berry detox water

Ideally, lemon should be an integral part of our daily meals. If your daily diet does not contain enough lemon, the easiest way is to use it in the daily intake of fruit infused waters. The goodness of lemon in the form of vitamin C plays a vital role in flushing out the toxins from your body. Packed with nourishing antioxidants, berries can significantly help in accelerating your weight loss regime. Drinking this interesting concoction for about 12-15 days in a row along with a healthy diet can give you the much-desired results for your weight loss.

Ingredients

- 1 cup fresh blueberries
- 1 cup fresh raspberries
- 1 sliced lemon
- 10-12 cups of water

Instructions

- Wash the berries. Ensure they are properly cleaned.
- Add the berries to an aqua blend basket along with lemon slices. Give it a mix.
- Pour water into the basket and mix all the ingredients well by stirring it.
- Leave the mixture in the basket for 3 hours before you could serve. The longer you store this concoction you are bound to get a richer flavor.
- Serve with ice cubes for that cooling effect.

Watermelon Rosemary Water

Avid dieters need to experiment more with tropical fruits like watermelon. More adventurous dieters would always want to add a bit of herbs in their detox waters. Rosemary can add a sweet smell to your drink, almost like a refreshing cocktail. The combined flavor of rosemary with watermelon can make for a brilliant combination while keeping your body hydrated. This delightful surprise can keep the boredom away when it comes to your detox diet. Anyone who thinks alcoholic drinks are the only way to enjoy should give this fantastic elixir a must try.

Ingredients

- 2 cups of watermelon (cubed and deseeded)
- 2 rosemary sprigs
- 2 tablespoons rose water
- 7-8 cups of water

Instructions

- Gently rub the rosemary sprigs in between your palms so it releases the flavor. Set aside in a bowl.
- Add cubed watermelon pieces to the infuser. Pour water, rose water, and stir it using a wooden spoon. Add the rosemary sprigs to it. Give it another stir
- Let the mixture stand for 2 hours and then serve. You can double up the quantity of the ingredients and store this drink the refrigerator for another day.

- Ensure to serve along with ice cubes.

Strawberry, Apple and Cinnamon drink for beautiful skin

One can never undermine the importance of drinking enough water to keep your skin clear and glowing. Dry skin, pimples, acne etc. can be reduced merely by drinking at least 7 – 8 glasses of water each day. To this routine, add a bit of antioxidants and you will have that youthful glow on your face that will leave you looking radiant. Strawberries and apples contain anti ageing agent like biotin, which works against sagging skin. Cinnamon on the other hand, helps in improving blood circulation and keeps you sugar cravings at bay. It is also often used in weight loss diets. Adding a dash of lemon zest to this drink can make it even more delightful.

- **Ingredients**

- 1 cup of fresh strawberries

- 1 medium sized apple (thinly sliced)

- 1 cinnamon stick

- Zest of one lemon

- 10-12 cups of water

Instructions

- Wash the strawberries properly.

- Add them to a large sized aqua basket. To this, add chopped apple slices, cinnamon and mix.

- Pour water, sprinkle some lemon zest and gently give the mixture a stir until it mixes well.

- Now leave this mixture in the refrigerator for a few hours for the infusion to take place. You can store this mixture for another day and consume as per your liking. Serve it chilled.

Anxiety reliever Pineapple Strawberry drink

The idea of a stress relieving magic potion may seem to be too good to be true. However, this next fruit infused recipe is sure to leave you pleasantly surprised with its results. Amidst the hectic schedule, office goers often stop by the canteen to grab a cup of coffee. While coffee could certainly seem like a stress reliever in the moment, excess amounts of it could be harmful to your health. A fruit infused stress-alleviating drink could be the perfect solution you may be looking for. High in anti oxidants, pineapple, and strawberries could leave you feeling refreshed for the rest of the day. Slight bit of apple cider vinegar could also help in weight loss.

Ingredients

- Half cup peeled and cubed pineapple
- 1 cup of strawberries
- 2 tablespoons of apple cider vinegar
- 7-8 cups of water
- 1 basil leaf

Instructions

- Wash the strawberries properly

- Take a large pitcher and add the washed strawberries to it. Now add pineapple, basil leaf and mix well.

- Pour water into the mixture. Add apple cider vinegar and give it a nice stir using a large spoon.

- Let it rest in the refrigerator for a few hours so the mixture gets infused well. Stronger flavors can be obtained if you leave it overnight. Serve chilled.

Blackberry and Sage water

The delectable combination of blackberries and sage can make this drink one of the most irresistible concoctions of all times. The spicy sage can leave you with a feeling of a full tummy while adding that much needed uniqueness to this drink. This purple colored drink can easily quench your thirst, while keeping you protected against acid imbalance, allergies and reduces menopausal symptoms. If you are feeling a little more adventurous, you can also try it with a dash of mint or cilantro leaves.

Ingredients

- 1 cup of fresh blackberries

- 4 sage leaves

- Few cilantro or mint leaves

- 8-10 cups of regular water

Instructions

- Wash the berries.

- Rub the sage leaves using both hands and set them aside.

- In a large vessel, add the berries, sage leaves, and cilantro and mix well. Pour water and keep stirring until it's mixed well.

- Transfer this mixture to an infuser bottle or a pitcher.

- Infusion process of this mixture will take at least a couple of hours this drink can be stored for another day in the refrigerator.

- Ensure to serve along with some ice cubes.

Kiwi lemonade

A delicious and juicy fruit like kiwi is one of the most ideal when it comes to making fruit infused waters. Having said that, kiwi may require a bit of more soaking so it could release the maximum flavors. The splash of green color and the tangy taste can turn a simple drink into a more delightful treat. Since it's not bitter like citrus skins, you can also use the rind for added flavor in your drinks. The tangy taste of kiwi and lemon can be balanced with a dash of honey and your drink is ready.

Ingredients

- 2 medium sized kiwis

- 1 sliced lemon

- 2-3 tablespoons of honey
- 7-8 cups of regular water

Instructions

- Wash the kiwis well and cut them into thin slices.
- Take a large pitcher and add the kiwi and lemon slices to it. Pour 8 cups of water, honey and stir well.
- Like mentioned earlier, the kiwis may take a bit longer to soak. Hence it's advisable to let this mixture stand for 4 hours before it's served.
- Ensure to add generous amounts of ice cubes while serving this drink.

Peach and Ginger infused cooler

I wonder if there is anything more pleasing than reading a book on a lazy Sunday evening alongside a peach and mint cooler. This concoction can easily uplift your mood while giving you a cooling effect. The tasty peach is an ideal snack for shedding those extra pounds. A single peach consists of merely 50 calories without any fat. Plus, it helps in keeping your skin healthy and hair loss at bay. A bit of mint along with some vanilla can enhance the flavor of this drink by a few notches. If you don't find fresh peaches, you can also use the frozen ones.

Ingredients

- 5 medium sized peaches
- 6-7 mint leaves
- Half a pod of vanilla
- 7-8 cups of water

Instructions

- Wash the peaches and slice them up using a sharp knife. Set aside.
- In a huge infuser, add the peaches, mint leaves and mix.
- Pour water into the infuser and stir it. Add a bit of vanilla and give it a stir again.
- This concoction takes about 2 hours to get infused. Store it in the refrigerator for a few hours.
- Serve chilled.

Peach and Ginger Water

Take the warmth of the ginger and the sweetness of the peaches, and you have an interesting drink that can quench your thirst without adding too many calories. The numerous health benefits of both peach and ginger makes it for a perfect health drink. It could contain as low as 40 calories per serving. You can add the peach and ginger skin to various deserts such as cakes, panacotta or ice creams for added flavor.

Ingredients

- 4 medium sized peaches
- 1 piece of ginger (2inch)
- 4 sprigs cilantro
- 7-8 cups of water

Instructions

- Wash the peaches and ginger properly. Peel the ginger and cut them into thin slices.
- Break the cilantro sprigs. Add them to a large infuser. Now add the sliced peaches, ginger and mix.
- Pour water to this mixture and stir.
- Let it stand for two hours before you are ready to serve. You can also strain this mixture before serving. Alternatively after consuming the drink you can also relish on the peach pieces.
- Add ice cubes.

Cucumber and Lavender Water

This drink can help in alleviating all types of indigestion issues, bloating, as well as dehydration. Cucumber, known for its anti-inflammatory properties can provide a huge relief for your tummy and help your body to rehydrate. The effect of lavender can aid in relieving anxiety or stress issues, while lending the drink a wonderful floral aroma. Adding mint to this drink can also ensure that you stay fresh throughout the day.

Ingredients

- 1 large cucumber
- 4-5 lavender leaves (fresh or packaged)
- 5 mint leaves
- 10-12 cups of water

Instructions

- Wash the cucumber and cut it into thin slices using a sharp knife.
- In a large container, add cucumber slices along with the lavender leaves. Gently rub the mint leaves using both hands and add them to the mix.
- Pour water and stir the drink using a large spoon.
- Now transfer this mixture to an infuser bottle and let the infusion process take place for about 2 hours. You can also refrigerate it overnight for better results.
- Make sure to always serve it chilled

Grapefruit, Mint & Ginger concoction

Grapefruits are widely known to increase blood circulation in the body and works as an anti-ageing factor. Regular use of grapefruits cannot only slow down the ageing process but also cures dry skin issues. Similarly, it is also known to boost the immune system thus keeping you protected against diseases. Most of our weekend hangouts leave us with a heavy hangover that takes a while to snap out of. This drink is exactly what you need to curb the hangover in merely a few minutes of you consuming the drink.

Ingredients

- 1 large cup of fresh grapefruit
- Half a cucumber
- 2 slices of ginger (2 inch)
- 4 mint leaves
- 1 small orange (peeled)
- 10-12 cups of water

Instructions

- Wash and peel the ginger. Wash the grapefruit properly. Peel and slice the cucumber.
- Take a large aqua blend basket and add the ginger slices, orange pieces, mint and grapefruit to it. Pour some water.
- Stir it well using a wooden spoon until it's mixed properly. Leave this mixture for three hours for it to release maximum flavors. Store it in the refrigerator if you would like.
- Serve with ice cubes.

Papaya and lime concoction

Papayas have found a place in a wide variety of cuisines all across the globe, especially Brazil and India. Papaya is packed with a high amount of minerals, copper, and potassium that can reduce fatigue. Copper is known to boost the connective tissues in the body and potassium can reduce the risk of heart attacks. Papaya and lime together can help in boosting your immune system to a large extent while adding delicious flavors to the drink.

Ingredients

- 1 small sized papaya (ripened)
- 2 small sized limes
- Half teaspoon of vanilla extract
- 7-8 cups water

Instructions

- Wash the papaya. Peel the skin off it and cut it into small sized cubes. Cut thin slices of lime using a sharp knife.
- Take a pitcher and add papaya and lime pieces to it. To this, add the vanilla extract and pour water.
- Ensure to stir this mixture well so it blends properly. You can also use a few berries to give it a tangy taste.
- Let this concoction stand for three hours for it to get perfectly infused. You can always store this drink in the

refrigerator for a day. Be generous with the ice cubes while serving.

Mango and Mint cooler

Don't fret about not being able to find a fully ripened mango. This drink can be made out of semi-ripened mangoes and still taste delicious. Mango is not only a delicious fruit but it's loaded with anti-oxidants. Also high in vitamin C, regular use of mango can play a vital role in the production of collagen, which is helpful in preventing the skin from sagging. The other health benefits of mango include reduction in cholesterol issues, prevention against cancer and works against night blindness. Mango and mint makes for a soul soothing combination especially when you are feeling tired.

Ingredients

- Medium sized mango
- 5 mint leaves
- 2 tablespoons of honey
- 7-8 cups of regular water

Instructions

- Wash, peel and cut the mango into thin slices.
- Take a large vessel and add the mango slices to it. To this, add mint leaves, honey and mix well.

- Pour water and give it a stir. This particular drink may need to be kept aside for three hours for the perfect infusion to take place.

- Serve chilled or use ice cubes.

Orange vanilla infused water

Orange combined with a dash of vanilla is an extremely healthy and a delectable concoction that can even be served in parties. This drink can be a huge hit among your loved ones and can be served alongside some ice cream. Oranges are perfect for uplifting your mood without adding too many calories to your drink. Vanilla on the other hand, not only adds an oomph to your detox water, but also hydrates your skin.

Ingredients

- 1 large sized orange
- 3/4 teaspoon vanilla extract
- 2 tablespoons honey
- 7-8 cups regular water

Instructions

- Peel the orange and set aside in a bowl. To this, add honey and vanilla extract. Mix well.

- Take a large infuser and fill it with some water. Add orange, honey and vanilla extract and give it a stir.

- Allow this mixture to stand for an hour. You can also make this drink a day ahead of the party and keep it ready for serving.

- Add ice cubes as per your liking.

Cucumber and Jalapeno drink

If you have been looking for a kickass detoxifier, this drink would be it. Slightly unusual combination of the cooling cucumber with spicy jalapeno chilies is for the experimental dieters. Cucumber acts as a deterrent for kidney or liver problems, while keeping the body away from ammonia. Jalapeno on the other hand can add an instant oomph to most food items and is also known to accelerate your body's metabolism. The spicy flavor of jalapeno chili can be adjusted according to your taste. You can also spruce up the drink by adding a dash of lemon to it.

Ingredients

- 1 medium sized cucumber
- 3 small sized jalapeno peppers
- 7-8cups of water
- Half a lemon

Instructions

- Wash the cucumber, jalapeno peppers, and lemon and cut them into thin slices.

- Take a vessel and add the above ingredients to it and mix well.

- Pour water and give it a good stir. Feel free to adjust the amount of jalapeno chilies used in the recipe.

- Serve chilled or add some ice cubes to the drink.

Pineapple and Thyme water

Tired of using the same old fruits for making detox drinks? You should try adding some herbs to make it interesting. Herbs can turn a simple detox drink into a flavorful and mouthwatering concoction you can't seem to get enough of. Pineapple contains a blood-thinning agent known as the bromelain, thereby reducing the risk of a heart stroke. Whereas thyme can provide abundant amount of iron required for your body to function well. It also alleviates inflammation and contains antibacterial properties. This sweet and herby drink is quick to make and is super delicious.

Ingredients

- 1 cup peeled cubed pineapple
- 1 sprig of thyme
- 1tablespoon honey
- 7-8 cups water

Instructions

- Rip the leaves of thyme and rub them slightly with your hand for it to release the maximum flavor. Put it in a

- bowl and add pineapple pieces and honey to it. Mix all the ingredients.

- Take a large infuser bottle and pour about 7-8 cups of water in it. Now add the mixture from the bowl, a spoonful of honey and stir for about a few seconds.

- Set this mixture aside for two hours so it gets infused well. If you can't seem to finish off the entire drink, store it up in the refrigerator for 24 hours.

- Serve in attractive glasses.

Cranberry and Rosemary drink

We all are visual creatures when it comes to food or drinks. The more attractive a drink looks. The more we are drawn to it. Some are so visual that they don't mind an attractive looking drink with a mediocre taste. Here's a drink that is almost picturesque as well as tasty. Cranberries are an ideal fruit to keep your immune system healthy while providing you enough nutrients at the same time. When you flavor up the sweet and tangy taste of cranberries with some aromatic rosemary, you get an amazing drink that can satiate your taste buds.

Ingredients

- 1 cup fresh cranberries
- 2 rosemary sprigs
- 1 medium sized apple
- 8-10 cups of water

Instructions

- Wash the cranberries and apple. Slice up the apples using a sharp knife.

- Rip the rosemary leaves for maximum flavor. Add all these ingredients together in a bowl and mix.

- Pour water in a large pitcher and add all the ingredients in the bowl to it. Stir it well using a large spoon.

- Infusion for this drink will take at least two hours. Store it up in the fridge overnight for a richer flavor.

- Serve chilled.

Cranberry, Orange & Bay leaf Cooler

If you are an avid fan of refreshing tangy concoctions, this drink is for you. There are different ways to transform seemingly boring detox water into a fancy one. The combination of cranberry and orange plays out beautifully in terms of flavors as well as the color. To add an herby aroma, you can experiment with bay leaf to lend a unique flavor to the drink. The phytonutrients present in cranberry ensures that it's packed with antioxidants and acts as an anti inflammatory agent.

Ingredients

- 1 cup of cranberries

- 2 medium sized oranges (peeled)

- 1 big bay leaf

- 7-8 cups of water

Instructions

- Wash the cranberries well. You can cut up the cranberries to bring out more flavors.

- Pour the water into a large container. To this, add the cranberries, orange pieces, and bay leaf and stir well. Mix all the ingredients properly using a large spoon.

- Add a generous amount of ice cubes to this mixture and leave it for infusion for two hours. Make this drink a day before the weekend so you can enjoy a cozy evening sipping on it. Store it overnight for 24 hours.

- Go generous with the amount of ice cubes while serving this drink.

Apple and Ginger concoction

Apples have a wider appeal in terms of its usage in several different foods. Besides its wide usage in desserts and juices due to the high fiber content, it has several medicinal properties too. However, you have to be extra careful about picking up the right kind of apples from the market. Always check the apples for any wax coating they may be laden with, as they may be sprayed with too many pesticides. Pick the ones that look naturally red and have a non-glossy finish. The fantastic combination of apple and ginger can be a great cure for cough too.

Ingredients

- 2 medium sized apples
- 2 ginger roots (2 inch)
- 3 tablespoons of honey
- 10-12 cups of water

Instructions

- Wash the apples properly. If you ended up buying the wax-coated apples by error, peel the skin off and cut them into thin slices. Similarly, peel the skin off the ginger roots and slice them up.

- Take some water in an infuser. To this, add the apple and ginger pieces. Mix them well.

- Add some honey to this drink and mix the ingredients well.

- Let it stand for two hours for the perfect infusion. Keep it in the fridge for a few more hours for a richer taste.

- Serve ice cubes with the drink.

Cherry and Mint infused Water

Going on a diet can often leave people with a sweet tooth craving for sugar. While cutting down refined sugar from your daily intake is important for weight loss, it can get difficult to control the craving. Cherries can add that much needed sweetness to your detox drink without adding excess calories to it. Cherry and mint can make for a spectacular drink without added preservatives and chemicals. The pepper minty taste of this drink will also give you instant refreshment after a long days work. Enjoy sipping it slowly by the poolside on a lazy afternoon.

Ingredients

- 1 cup of fresh cherries
- 5 mint leaves
- Half cinnamon stick
- 7-8 cups of water

Instructions

- Wash the cherries and cut them into two halves if you wish. Doing this will release maximum flavor and make your drink more relishing.
- Rip off the mint leaves and give them a gentle rub using your hands.
- Take a large pitcher and add the cherries, mint and cinnamon stick to it. Pour water and keep stirring it slowly until all the ingredients get mixed well.
- Leave it aside for 2 hours for the flavors to get infused. To get a richer flavor, store this drink in the fridge for about 24 hours.
- Add ice cubes while serving.

Mango & lemon grass infused Water

How about a lip smacking and thirst quenching cocktail minus the excess calories? It's a drink that is rich in flavors and at the same time detoxifies your body. Using lemongrass for your detox waters can bring about an X-factor to an otherwise plain drink. Also, lemon grass can be grown in your private nursery without needing anything else besides a rich soil, strategically placed pot so as to derive sunlight and lots of water. It helps in curbing excess hunger; cures water retention, and also acts as an antioxidant that can prevent wrinkles from appearing on your skin.

Ingredients

- 2 medium sized mangoes
- 1 stalk of lemon grass (husk removed)
- 5 strawberries
- 10-12 cups of water

Instructions

- Wash, peel and slice the mangoes into small cubes. Similarly, wash the strawberries and cut them into two halves. Set aside in a bowl. Bash the lemon grass slightly so it releases a richer flavor. Add it to the bowl and mix well.

- In a large aqua blend basket, add the ingredients from the bowl along with some water. Stir continuously for about a minute. Ensure all ingredients are mixed well.

- Let this concoction stand for three hours before it could be served. Doing this will allow the infuse process to take place. Refrigerate overnight for better taste and flavor.

- Add 3-4 ice cubes per serving.

Blackberry and Lemon grass infused water

There's something nostalgic about sipping on a rustic drink from a cool pitcher on a weekend campout, reminiscing all the pleasant memories of your life. As relaxing as it sounds, this drink can soothe your senses in minutes and leave you feeling peaceful. This drink could your perfect savior on a blistery summer morning. You can also combine this drink with your daily cup of green iced tea. The aroma of lemon grass, tangy taste of blackberry, cooling cucumber and revitalizing green tea could be just what you need to kick start your day with a bang.

Ingredients

- 1 cup of blackberries
- 1 small sized cucumber
- 1 stalk of lemon grass (de-husked)
- 8-10 cups of water

Instructions

- Wash the blackberries and cucumber. Slice up the cucumber using a sharp knife.

- Bash the lemon grass stalk so it gives out a rich aroma.

- Fill some water in a vessel. To this, add the blackberries, cucumber, and bashed lemon grass and give it a stir until all ingredients are mixed well.

- Transfer this mixture to an infuser bottle and let it stand for 2 hours. You can serve this drink along with some ice cubes after it has been infused well. Alternatively you can store it up to 24 hours in the fridge.

Raspberry Peach and Kiwi water

Today more and more people are education themselves about the side effects of excess refined sugar in their diet. This awareness is helping in ensuring that people cut down fizzy and sugary drinks from their diet. Fruit infused waters especially made using citrusy fruits like raspberry and kiwi are becoming a huge hit among youngsters. Raspberry, kiwi and peach make for a glamorous looking drink that contains all the qualities of a health drink. This drink tastes slightly sweetish without having to add any sugar. Adding a bit of cinnamon to this drink also helps in accelerating weight loss.

Ingredients

- 1 cup fresh or packaged raspberries

- 2 small peaches

- 2 medium sized kiwis

- Half a stick of cinnamon

- 10-12 cups of water

Instructions

- Wash the raspberries, cut them into two halves if you wish. Wash the peaches, kiwis and cut them up into slices.

- Take a large pitcher and fill it up with water. To this, add all the fruits, cinnamon stick and stir until the ingredients are mixed well.

- Let it stand for three hours. If you wish, you can refrigerate this drink for another day. It will bring out maximum flavors and make your drink even more enjoyable.

- Serve this drink along with ice cubes on top.

Lime and Tarragon detox water

Not a lot of people seem to develop a taste for Tarragon that easily. However, if you use this herb in moderation and not let it get overpowering, you are bound to get an interesting blend of flavors. Tarragon is generally used alongside citrusy fruits as it works well with them. Slightly anise like in taste, tarragon is best infused with lime. If you have never tried tarragon in your detox water, it's about time you should try it. This ultra refreshing spa water will also ensure that you stay away from fizzy drinks.

Ingredients

- 2 medium sized limes
- 1/2 cup fresh tarragon leaves
- 2 tablespoons honey
- 7-8 cups of water

Instructions

- Wash and cut the limes into thin slices.
- Slightly bash the tarragon leaves for it to release maximum flavor.
- Fill up an infuser bottle with some water. Throw in the tarragon leaves. Add lime slices to it along with some honey and stir well for about a minute.
- Let this concoction stand for two to three hours for the infusion to take place. Keep aside some water in the refrigerator so you can sip on it later.
- Serve along with some ice cubes.

Banana Honey and Basil infused water

Bananas may seem like an odd choice for making fruit infused waters for some, but once you give it a try, you may want to use it regularly. A lot of people think consuming bananas always leads to weight gain, however that's not true. When consumed in moderation, bananas can do wonders to your skin and health. They are high in potassium and are widely known to help proper digestion of food. Honey and banana can both keep your skin hydrated for a long time. This sweetish drink with a slightly herby taste of basil is enough to keep your hungers pangs in control.

Ingredients

- 1 large semi-ripened banana
- 2 tablespoons honey
- 2-3 basil leaves
- 7-8 cups of water

Instructions

- Peel the bananas and cut them into slices. Set the slices aside in a bowl. To this, add some honey. Gently bash the basil leaves and add them to the bowl. With the help of a spoon, mix all the ingredients well.

- Fill up a pitcher with some water. Transfer all the ingredients from the bowl to the pitcher and give it a stir using a large spoon.

- This mixture may take at least two hours to infuse. For better results, store it up in refrigerator for 24 hours.

- Serve chilled.

Banana Pineapple and Mint infused water

If you did end up liking the above-mentioned banana drink, you are going to love this one too. Here's a concoction that combines the hunger satiating properties of banana, the vitamin packed pineapple and the freshness of mint. As nutritious as this drink sounds, it's pretty rich in taste too. Although you have to avoid the use of extra ripened bananas as it may increase the sugar content of your drink. The fruits used to make this drink will also supply a good amount of dietary fiber to your body which necessary for proper digestion.

Ingredients

- 1 large sized semi-ripened banana
- 1 cup peeled and diced pineapple
- 1 sprig of mint
- 12 cups of water

Instructions

- Peel the banana and cut it into thin slices using a sharp knife.
- In a separate bowl, add the sliced banana, pineapple and slightly bashed mint leaves. Mix them together.
- Take about 12 cups of water in an aqua blend basket. To this, add all the ingredients from the bowl and keep stirring until all ingredients are mixed well.

- A minimum span of two hours is needed for this drink to get infused well. For enhanced flavor, try storing it up in the fridge overnight.

- Ensure to always serve this drink chilled.

Banana Strawberry & Cardamom infused water

Here's another magical recipe that you wish you had tried your hands on earlier. Adding strawberry to your banana infused water makes this drink super tasty. Strawberries add a beautiful pinkish color to the drink while giving it a slightly tangy taste. Then we have cinnamon that can make the drink easily appeal to your senses and help the detoxification process too. Cardamoms are easily available in the market and you can stock them up to one year in the refrigerator. Just ensure to keep them away from catching moisture.

Ingredients

- 1 medium sized banana
- 1 cup fresh strawberries
- 2 cardamom cloves
- 10 cups of water

Instructions

- Peel the banana and chop it using a sharp knife. Wash the strawberries thoroughly and slice them into two halves. Add these two ingredients to a bowl.

- Slightly pound the cardamoms for releasing its flavor. Now add it to the bowl and mixed all the ingredients using a spoon.

- Take a large pitcher and pour some water into it. Now transfer the ingredients from the bowl into the pitcher and stir continuously for about one minute.

- Let this mixture stand for a minimum of three hours for a richer taste. You can choose to store this mixture in the fridge for 12 hours for a perfectly infused drink.

- Don't forget to add ice cubes while serving.

Guava and Mango infused water

Guava is another fruit that most people don't think of adding in their daily dose of detox water. The idea of using a fruit like guava may seem slightly boring to you but when you combine it with citrusy fruits, it makes for a delightful drink. Mango too works well with guava. Adding a spoonful of honey to this drink will only enhance the flavor and give it a nice aroma. You can alternatively add a clove of cardamom too if you would like. High in antioxidants and vitamin C, little do people know that guava repairs dry skin too.

Ingredients

- 2 medium sized guavas
- 1 semi-ripened small sized mango
- 1 tablespoon honey
- 7-8 cups of water

Instructions

- Wash the guavas and mango and chop them into small cubes. Put these pieces in a bowl.

- Add some honey into the bowl and mix well using a spoon. Be sure to blend the mixture well.

- Take some water in a large vessel. Transfer the ingredients from the bowl to the vessel and stir properly. Pour this mixture into an infuser bottle.

- To make this drink more flavorful, let it stand for three hours or store it in the fridge overnight. Doing this will enhance the flavor of the drink.

- Add some ice cubes and serve this drink in attractive glasses.

Passion fruit Sage and honey infused water

Highly fragrant, delightful looking and citrusy, passion fruit can become an instant favorite when it comes to making your own detox water. Most passion fruit lovers can't seem to get enough of their regular dose of passion fruit juice. Adding them to your detox water can provide you a huge motivation to start going on a healthy diet. For all those who are craving to give their diets a cheat day can easily satisfy their sweet tooth by consuming this detox water. The spicy taste of sage and the subtle aroma of honey can make you addicted to this drink

Ingredients

- 2 medium sized passion fruit
- 1 sprig of sage
- 1 tablespoon honey
- 7-8 cups water

Instructions

- Take the skin off of the passion fruit and dice them up using a kitchen knife.
- Slightly bash the sage leaves for an enhanced flavor.
- In a large infuser bottle, throw in the bashed sage leaves, cubed passion fruit, honey and mix using a large spoon. Pour some water and give this mixture a good stir.
- The infusion for this drink may take up to 3 hours. The more time you store it in the fridge, the richer this drink shall taste.
- Always serve with 3-4 ice cubes on top.

Passion fruit Rosemary and Chia Water

The citrusy passion fruit can taste even better with a spoonful of chia seeds added to it. Chia seeds can be considered to be one of the super foods that can instantly providing a cooling effect to your body. Easily available in the stores and absolutely inexpensive, chia seeds once soaked can form a thin gelatin like layer around them just like tomato seeds. The sweetish fragrance of rosemary blends perfectly well with the juicy passion fruit, thereby creating a magical drink. Just ensure to avoid over usage of chia seeds so it does not overpower the taste of passion fruit.

Ingredients

- 2 Medium sized passion fruit
- 1 Tablespoon chia seeds
- 1 Sprig of rosemary
- 10 cups of regular water

Instructions

- Peel the skin off the passion fruit and slice them up into small sized cubes using a kitchen knife.
- You can either soak the chia seeds half an hour in advance for them to fluff up, or directly throw in some during the infusion process. Rip the leaves of the rosemary sprig and gently rub it with your hand to release its aroma.
- Fill up an infuser bottle with some water. To this, add the passion fruit slices, some chia seeds, rosemary leaves and keep stirring until it gets mixed well.
- Letting this mixture stand for at least 3 hours will ensure proper infusion to take place. Store it up if you would like for another 12 hours for a perfect taste.
- Serve chilled.

Passion fruit and Kiwi infused water

A kickass combination of passion fruit along with some kiwi can be truly energizing. Not only does it make for a glamorous looking drink, but also it can get you relaxed in minutes after consuming it. Both are extremely juicy fruits that can ensure a clear skin and better blood circulation. You can add any herb you would like to make this drink extra flavorful but using a clove of cardamom seems like a perfect addition. If you prefer a slightly sweetish taste, you can also add a spoonful of honey to this lovely concoction.

Ingredients

- 2 small sized passion fruit
- 2 small sized kiwis
- 2 small cardamom cloves
- 7-8 cups of regular water

Instructions

- Take the skin off the passion fruit using a small knife or a peeler. Cut the passion fruit and kiwis into thin slices. Set them aside in a bowl.

- Slightly pound the cardamom cloves for releasing its aroma. Add them to the bowl. If you prefer the cardamom without its skin, you can use just the seeds.

- Fill up a large glass pitcher with about 8 cups of water. Add the ingredients on the bowl to it and stir well using a large spoon that can reach the end of the bottom.

- Infusion process for this drink will take a minimum of 3 hours. Give it another 12 hours for an enhanced flavor and taste.

- Use a generous amount of ice cubes while serving.

Passion fruit, Tender Coconut and Vanilla water

Passion fruit and vanilla martini has been gaining a lot of popularity in recent times. While an alcoholic drink can be truly enjoyable at times, sipping on some detox water using the same combination tastes just as great. This combination can make for a great evening drink, especially with the addition of tender coconut pieces. While vanilla can add a great flavor to the drink, tender coconut will give you that ice cold effect and leave you feeling with a full tummy feeling. You can also gorge on the passion fruit and tender coconut slices after you have consumed the drink.

Ingredients

- 2 medium sized passion fruit
- 1 cup tender coconut pieces
- 1 teaspoon vanilla extract
- 12 cups of water

Instructions

- Peel the skin off the passion fruit using a small knife. Cut it into small 1-inch cubes and set them aside in a bowl.

- Add the tender coconut pieces, some vanilla extract and mix well using a spoon.

- Take some water in a large vessel and fill it up with some water. Transfer the ingredients from the ball into the vessel and keep storing continuously for about a minute. Transfer this mixture into infuser bottles for storage.

- Let this concoction stand for 3 hours for the infusion process to take place. Overnight storage of this drink in the fridge is sure to make it more flavorful.

- Always serve cold or add ice cubes while serving.

Passion fruit, Papaya and Mint infused water

Passion fruit being slightly tangy in taste, you can sometimes team it up with a subtle flavored fruit like papaya. If you are a true passion fruit lover, you may not want another fruit to overpower its flavor. This combination will balance both the flavors while you can relish on the fruit chunks after you finish off the drink. Mint is always a favorite among dieters when it comes to their detox waters as it gives a fresh flavor to the drink while also helping in clear any digestion issues.

Ingredients

- 2 medium sized passion fruit

- 1 small papaya

- 2 sprigs of mint leaves

- 10-12 cups of water

Instructions

- Take the skin off the passion fruit as well as papaya using a kitchen knife. Cut them into small 1-inch cubes and set them aside.

- Slightly rub the mint leaves in order to get more flavors off them.

- Take some water in an infuser bottle. Add the papaya and passion fruit cubes to it along with the mint leaves. Now cover the lid of the bottle and shake it for about a minute so all the ingredients get mixed properly.

- Let this mixture stand for 2 hours for the infusion process to take place. Place it in the refrigerator for a much flavorful drink.

- Serve in an attractive glass and add some ice cubes.

Passion fruit Blueberry and cinnamon water

A lot of people with dry skin tend to go berserk with beauty products to keep their skin hydrated. While using the right moisturizer or any other beauty product can certainly do you some good, it's also important to keep the body hydrated from inside. Adding citrusy fruits to your daily diet ensures a proper blood flow thereby keeping your skin hydrated. The more hydrated your skin remains, the better its chances of preventing it from getting dry. Instead of spending a fortune on beauty products, you can use natural fruits like passion fruit and blueberries to your diet.

Ingredients

- 2 medium sized passion fruit
- 1 cup of fresh blueberries
- 1 cinnamon stick
- 1 tablespoon honey
- 12 cups of water

Instructions

- For starters, you need to take the skin off the passion fruit using a sharp knife. Cut them into small pieces.
- Wash the blueberries. Add both the fruits in a bowl. To his, add honey and mix well.
- Fill up some water in a large aqua blend casket. Transfer the ingredients form the bowl to this casket and give it a stir. Add the cinnamon stick and stir again.
- You can also transfer this mixture to an infuser bottle and let it stand for three for it to get infused well. Alternatively, you can choose to store it overnight in the fridge for a better taste.
- Serve chilled.

Lychee and pineapple infused water

Who doesn't love lychees? This tropical fruit is easily available in the markets now. Fresh or packaged, it can add a great flavor to a detox drink. Extremely rich in phytonutrients, antioxidants and vitamin B-complex, lychee can also be a delightful fruit to gorge on. This tiny looking fruit is also loaded with high amount of nutrients that can be useful for your bodily functions. The zesty pineapple brings a sweet and tangy taste to this drink and leaves you feeling satiated. A few leaves of thyme or sage can make this mixture more interesting and keep the boredom out of the window when it comes to detox drinks.

Ingredients

- 12 medium sized lychees
- 1 cup of cubed pineapple
- 1 sprig of thyme leaves
- 12 cups of water

Instructions

- Peel the skin off the lychees using your hands. Remove the seed and cut them into two halves. Take a bowl and add the pineapple cubes and lychees to it.
- Rip the thyme leaves apart and gently rub them in between your palms. Doing this will bring out maximum flavor

- Fill up a large pitcher with some water. Transfer the ingredients from the bowl to it. Throw in the thyme leaves and stir it for about a minute.

- Let the mixture stand for at least three hours for a better flavor. For a richer flavor, store this drink in the fridge for another 12 hours and you are ready to serve.

- Use loads of ice cubes while serving.

Lychee Orange and chia seeds water

Imagine sipping on the most rejuvenating drink in a spa while enjoying the nature. This ultra refreshing drink is perfect for a hot sunny day. While it is blistering hot outside, you can feel relaxed and put your feet up without having a thing to worry about. A spectacular combination of lychee, chia seeds and orange can alleviate the excess heat in the body. The punch of lychee when combined with the zesty orange can revitalize your senses instantly. The unique flavor of this fruit punch is sure to leave a lovely aftertaste in your mouth the entire day.

Ingredients

- 10 medium sized lychees
- 1 medium sized orange
- 1 tablespoon of chia seeds
- 12 cups of water

Instructions

- You can easily rip apart the lychee skin using your bare hands. After peeling the skin off, remove the seeds and cut them into two halves. Set aside in a bowl. Peel the orange and add it to the bowl.

- In a large vessel, pour some water. To this, add the ingredients in the bowl. Throw in some chia seeds and keep stirring until it's mixed well.

- Allow this concoction to stand for three hours for a flavorful drink. Best results can be obtained by storing up this drink in the fridge for 24 hours.

- Serve chilled.

Lychee and ginger infused water

This combination may seem unusual at the first go, but we strongly recommend you to try it. The ginger root can bring a spicy taste to the drink, which is exactly what you may need during a wintery evening. When its winters, you don't want to gorge on too many cooling fruits as it could give you a cold. The cooling effect of lychee gets well balanced by adding some ginger to it. It may sound like an out of the box drink, but it may end up becoming your favorite and also provide you with the medicinal properties of ginger especially in winters. Ginger is also widely used for weight loss drinks.

Ingredients

- 12 large sized lychees
- 2 ginger roots (1 inch each)

- 1 tablespoon honey

- 12 cups of regular water

Instructions

- Wash the lychees and rip its skin apart. Cut them into two halves using a kitchen knife.

- Wash the ginger roots properly. Ensure it's not muddled with soil. Peel its skin off using a peeler. Cut into thin slices.

- To a large pitcher, add some water along with the above ingredients and mix well. Add a spoonful of honey and give it a good stir.

- Allow this mixture to get infused for about three hours. You can also transfer this liquid in an infuser bottle and store it in the ridge overnight.

- Serve along with some ice cubes on top.

Dragon Fruit coconut water and basil concoction

While we all agree that taste matters the most rather than how the food or the drink looks, let's admit it, I would prefer a good looking drink. Dragon fruit makes the drink visually stunning while adding its refreshing and unique flavor to it. This pinkish magenta colored drink is something everyone wants to gorge on at house parties. Since kids are more visual, they would enjoy this drink the most. Basil is used in several from of cuisines to enhance the flavor the food. Using Basil detox water helps in cleansing your digestive tract and increases blood circulation.

Ingredients

- 2 medium sized dragon fruits
- 2 large cups of coconut water
- 6 basil leaves
- 12 cups of water

Instructions

- Using a small knife, make a long slit on the skin of the passion fruit. Now rip off the skin using your hands and remove the fruit. Cut it into small cubes and set it aside.

- Take an infuser bottle and fill it up with some water. To this, add some coconut water, basil leaves, passion fruit cubes and close the lid of the bottle. Now give it a nice shake so all the ingredients in the bottle mix well.

- Allow this mixture to get infused in the bottle for a couple of hours. Store this bottle in the fridge in case you want a richer taste.

- Don't forget to add a generous amount of ice cubes while serving this drink.

Dragon fruit lemonade

Are you planning on picking up lemonade bottles from Wal-Mart for that football match you are planning to invite your friends for? Soda based drinks certainly double up your enjoyment, but one doesn't realize how badly it affects your health. Instead let's try a detox drink that could be just as refreshing, healthy and absolutely delicious too. Lemonade can provide that instant splash of energy you need while proving to be extremely healthy for your body. You can add a bit of pomegranate and add a more sweetish taste to the drink. Dragon fruit lemonade is not something that has been experimented enough in spite of its palette soothing taste.

Ingredients

- 2 medium sized dragon fruit
- 2 medium sized lemons
- 1 small cup of pomegranate (peeled)
- 12 cups of water

Instructions

- Rip the skin off the dragon fruit by making a slit on it using a knife. It's easy to pull apart the skin using your hands. Now cut the passion fruit into small cubes.
- Wash the lemons and cut them into thin slices
- Add water to a large pitcher. Throw in the dragon fruit pieces along with the lemons. Add pomegranate seeds and use a large spoon to stir this mixture. Ensure to stir it for a while so all ingredients get mixed properly.
- Serve chilled.

Dragon Rosemary and Watermelon drink

The very attractive looking dragon fruit is not just a visual treat but also contains several health benefits. The cactus like skin of the dragon fruit resembles almost like a mythical dragon, hence the name "dragon fruit". This tropical fruit can be found in abundance especially in Asian countries as well as South America. Regular use of dragon fruit in your diet helps in maintaining your cardiovascular health provides you ample amount of fiber fights blood sugar issues and lowers the signs of ageing. Watermelon and dragon are both high in their antioxidant properties and make for a delectable drink.

Ingredients

- 2 medium sized dragon fruit
- 1 large cup of watermelon (skin removed and cubes)
- 1 sprig of rosemary
- 12 cups of water

Instructions

- Take the skin off the dragon fruit. Due to its thin skin, you can easily peel it by making a slit. Now cut the fruit into small 1-inch cubes.
- To a bowl, add the watermelon and dragon fruit pieces and set aside. Slightly rub the rosemary leaves to release its flavor and add it to the bowl. Mix well using a spoon.

- Add some water to a large pitcher. Add the mixture from the bowl and using a large spoon keep stirring it until mixed well.

- Let this concoction stand for about three hours for the infusion to take place. If you want to store this drink keep it in the refrigerator overnight. This will also enhance its flavor.

- Serve chilled.

Pomegranate and Cucumber drink

Staying hydrated does not need to be boring or that you have to drink gallons of regular water. Ideally, your water intake needs to be at least 6-8 glasses for your body to function well. But why make this a boring routine when you can use interesting mix of pomegranate and cucumber for your detox drink. Pomegranate is known to have one of the highest amounts of antioxidants content among fruits. These red pearls are extremely beneficial in getting rid of any tummy issues or bloating. By combining the sweet juice taste of pomegranate and the cooling cucumber, you get a great summer drink.

Ingredients

- 2 cups of pomegranate (skin removed)

- 1 medium sized cucumber

- Zest of one large lemon

- 10-12 cups of water

Instructions

- Wash the cucumber and cut it into thin slices.

- In a bowl, add the pomegranate, cucumber slices, lemon zest and mix using a spoon.

- Pour some water in a large infuser bottle. To this, add the ingredients from the bowl. Close the lid of the bottle and shake it for a few seconds so the concoction gets mixed well.

- Serve chilled

Pomegranate Ginger and Limewater

Planning an all girl's night out on a wintery evening? Ditch that cola for this super tasty detox drink without adding excess calories. This perfect thirst quencher is an ideal choice on a cold evening surrounded by friends. The sweet taste of pomegranate along with some juicy lime and spicy ginger will make you want to sip on it the whole day.

Ingredients

- 2 cups of pomegranate (peeled)

- 1 two-inch ginger root

- 1 medium sized lime

- 12 cups of water

Instructions

- Wash the ginger root and lime properly and cut them into thin slices. Set them aside in a bowl.

- Add pomegranate to the bowl and mix using a spoon.

- Fill up a pitcher with regular water. Now transfer the ingredients from the bowl and give it a good stir using a wooden spoon.

- Now that your mixture is ready, you need to allow it to stand for 3 hours. For a better taste, leave it overnight in the fridge.

- Serve along with ice cubes.

Conclusion

Thank you for purchasing the book.

You have gathered all the knowledge that is required for a person who is now ready to start using fruit infused water. It may seem difficult to shift to something new at the beginning, but the zesty flavors of the fruit in the water will help in keeping you healthy and energetic. You have been given numerous recipes that you could use!

Keep your refrigerator stocked with jars of different types of fruit infused water! I hope you found this book helpful!

Made in the USA
Las Vegas, NV
27 November 2021